KATIE NOT-AFRAIDY
A Story About Conquering Childhood Anxiety

WRITTEN BY: GINA & DELILAH PERKINS
ILLUSTRATED BY: KRISTINA YU

Dedication & Thanks

We would like to dedicate this book
in loving memory of Mr. Mark Silverman, who touched thousands upon thousands of children's lives in his 35 year career as a teacher and counselor. Not only did Mark help each child find their inner Truth Queen/King, but he instilled within them the timeless virtue of being "kinder than necessary."

A special thank you to our unicorn editor,
Kimberly Graves

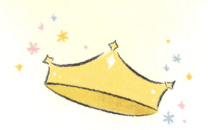

Hi!

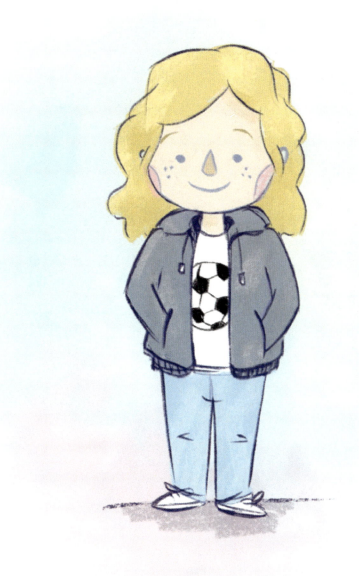

My name is Katie Not-Afraidy,
and I'm a really awesome kid.
Read along with me, you will
be glad you did.

I'm nine years old
and in third grade.
I enjoy doing lots of things
like most kids my age.

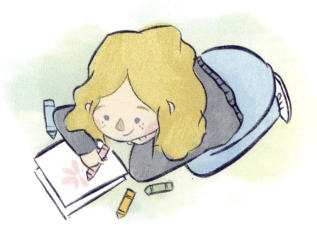

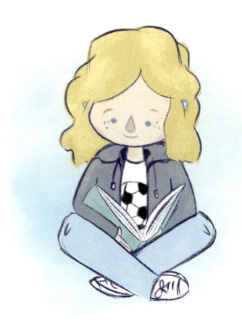

I play sports, write songs,
create art, and play games.
I also love to read books
in my favorite calmplace—
stories about animals, heroes,
shipwrecks and space.

I want to be a veterinarian
or maybe take care of
dolphins in a giant aquarium.
There isn't an animal
that I would turn away,
my cat and three dogs
are all here to stay.

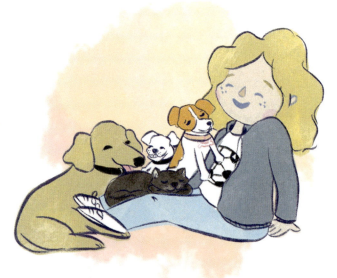

I must mention that I'm a big sister too.
My sister is 6 and playing together
is something we love to do.

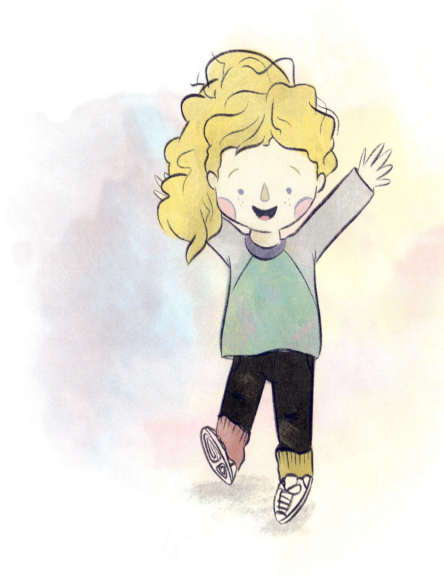

I can admit it is sometimes hard
to share my toys with her,
but she's my truest friend
of that I am sure.

I'm just a normal kid who's creative,
compassionate, generous, and smart.
I'm most proud of the ways kindness
flows from my heart.

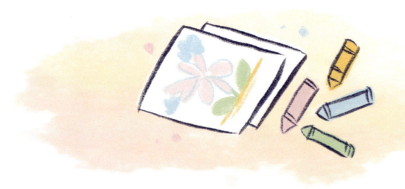

I include others on the playground
and pass encouraging words all around.

I use good manners and always help my teachers.
I'm a loyal friend, and I respect all creatures.

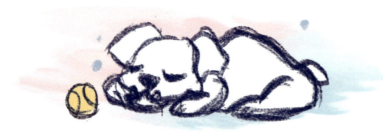

**What are some of the things
that make you most proud of you?**

I'm sure your list is super long too!

Write down some of the things that make you most proud of you on page 20.

My mom and dad tell me that I'm also incredibly brave.
It's hard for me to believe, because I'm often afraid.

I have really big worries
filling my head with bad stories.

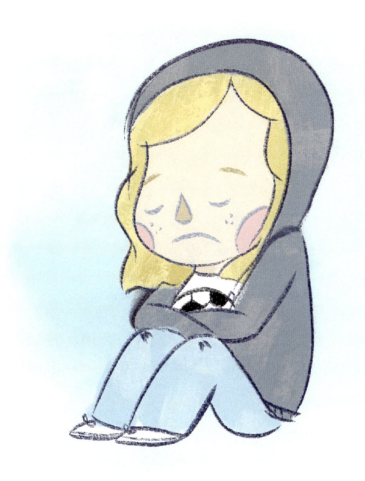

This makes me feel different
than other kids I know,
because my brain seems to be busier
than theirs' ever show.

The worries are like monsters that live inside my brain.
They mostly come out at night, and they fill me with shame.

They're loud, distracting, and keep me awake.
They tell big lies that make my chest ache.

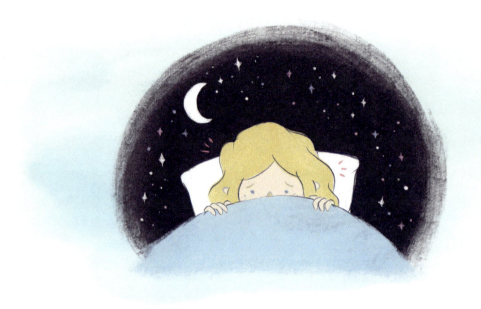

My mom tells me that worries are normal,
that some can even be healthy,
but my kind of worry is called anxiety.

Anxiety makes it hard for me to sleep at night
and tells me that I'm just not quite right.

If I want to go to a friend's house to play,
anxiety tells me that I won't be okay.

So then I'll stay home where I feel safe,
but that makes me feel sad because
I'm missing playdates.

In my house my mom has anxiety too.
She listens to my worries and
cheers me up when I'm blue.

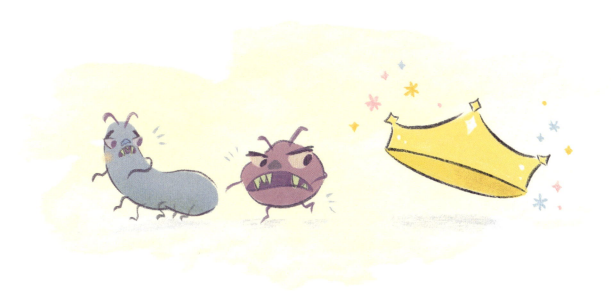

She helps me to understand
the battle inside my brain.
"You have a Truth Queen and
Story Bugs," she tries to explain.

My Truth Queen always tells me the truth.
She reminds me of my courage and acts like a sleuth.

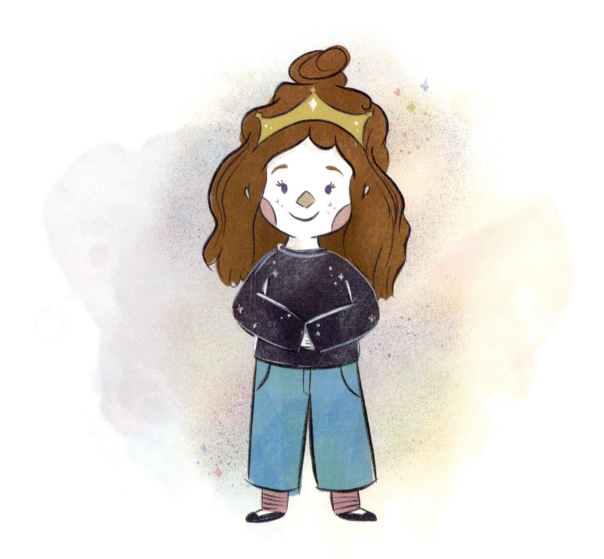

She points out all the times I have been strong
and shows me that I've been brave all along.

My Truth Queen reassures me that
monsters aren't living under my bed,
and that I have the power to push
that thought right out of my head.

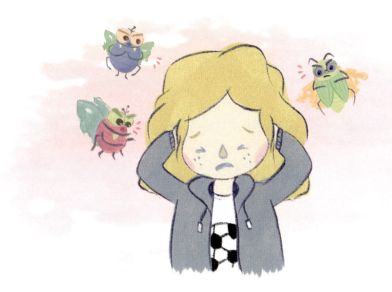

The Story Bugs are creepy, scary and mean.
They want me to ignore the wise Truth Queen.

These Bugs fill my head with lies
and once they get started
they keep growing in size.

The more attention I give them
the louder they get,
and the louder they get
the more that I fret.

The Story Bugs tell me that monsters are real,
and they don't care at all about how I feel.

**Do you have any Story Bugs
living inside your brain?**
Do they tell you the same
lies again and again?

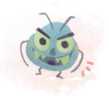

Turn to page 21, and write down any Story Bugs that you might have.

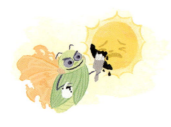

Sometimes the Story Bugs
sneak up just like a ninja attack.
They karate chop my mood
turning my sunny day black.

It actually hurts
so achy in my tummy.
My chest gets heavy,
and my head feels crummy.

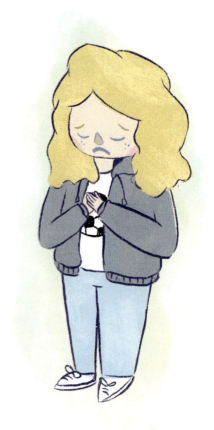

Other times the Story Bugs
slowly run through my mind
or hide in a corner just waiting to find
a worry to make me all dizzy inside.

The Story Bugs want
to knock me off my feet,
but I'm not going to be
that easy to defeat.

Thankfully, I've learned I can chase the Story Bugs away!
I can make them grow quieter and smaller each day.

I can stand up to them and show them who's boss!
Right outta my head all those lies get tossed.

When I am honest and tell others just how I feel,
the Story Bug lies feel less and less real.

The truth is I used to be kind of embarrassed of my anxiety.
It didn't seems like any other kids were quite like me.

For awhile I tried to just hold it all in,
but it grew and it grew; more talking just had to begin.

I started to talk to others about it
and that's when the Story Bugs started to quit.

I learned tools to chase those Story Bugs away.
I'll teach them to you, so don't go away.

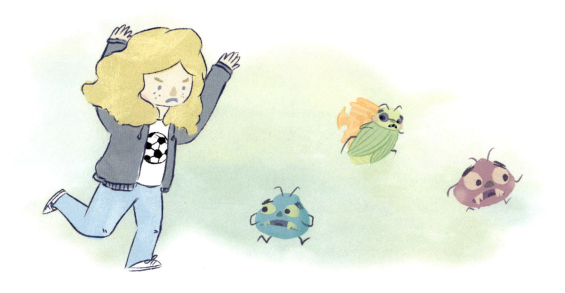

One way that I chase the Story Bugs away
is to take a deep breath and find a calm place to lay.

Closing my eyes helps me to calm down—
breathing in through my nose and out through my mouth.

I take a deep breath in while I slowly count to three,
and then hold it for two seconds and start to feel free.

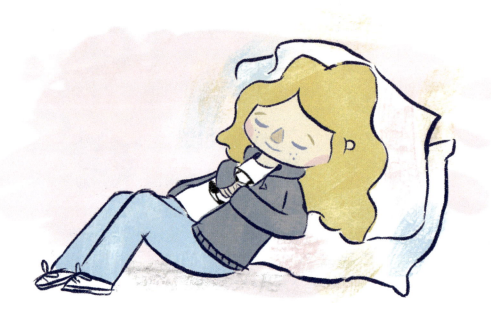

I finally exhale for a slow count of five,
and notice the Story Bugs shrinking in size.

I repeat this as many times as I need
until the Truth Queen's voice begins taking the lead.

When my anxiety makes me feel jittery and nervous inside,
deep breaths and the Truth are my calming guides.

If I have a worry I think of too often,
I put it in my worry box as a precaution.

Just putting my worries on paper helps me a lot.
It helps get my stomach out of a knot.

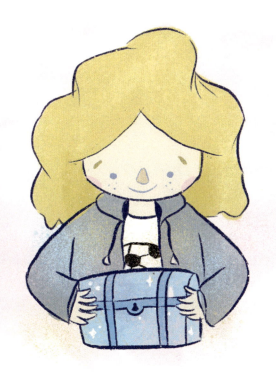

The worry box is where I can lock my worries away,
so I don't have to focus on them for that day.

Turn to page 22 for your very own mini worry box template.

Another thing that I find really helps
is to draw pictures of my worries
and pictures of myself.

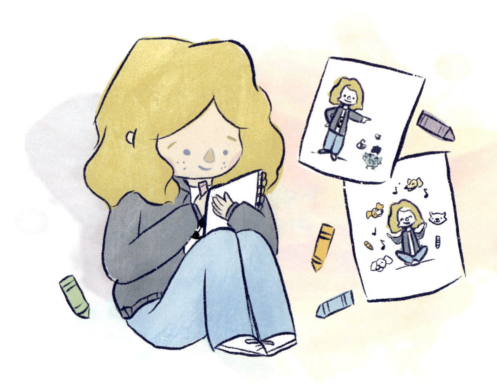

I draw my worries so small
and myself so tall
as a reminder that I am enough
to conquer them all.

Often when I get in bed at night,
the Story Bugs will all start to take flight.
I put on meditations or music for kids.
Bedtime story podcasts also have some help to give.

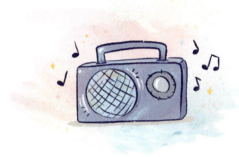

Music and stories
take my mind off the worries.
They set my imagination in motion,
almost like giving my Truth Queen
a magic truth potion!

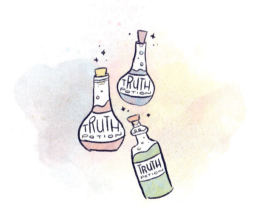

Every once in a while when music doesn't help,
I decide to have a nice talk with myself.
I know it sounds silly, but it does the trick.
I tell myself "I'm going to be okay!"
and I feel better quick.

These tools are all there in my anxiety toolbox.
If you try them you will find that they totally rock.

Some days you may get it right on the very first try,
and other days it may take some work
to tell the worries good-bye.

There is no right way to get through anxiety,
you just have to find what works
and simply believe.

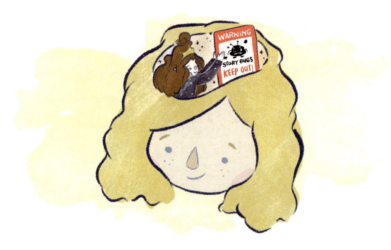

Just like me, your anxiety isn't who you are
and it will not win.
The Story Bugs have no power
when your Truth Queen charges in.

She is a part of you
your very own voice.
The bravest part of your soul
making a really bold choice.

Trust that you can do this. You can and you will.
The Story Bugs have no power in the lies that they spill.

My parents are right, I am brave and so are you!
There is nothing that we cannot do.

We are perfect just the way we are.
No matter how our brains work
we were born to be stars.

We are the heroes of our stories
our own Truth Queens and Kings.
Our anxiety won't stop us from being
who we were created to be.

I am Katie Not-Afraidy and I have anxiety,
but anxiety doesn't have me (or you.)

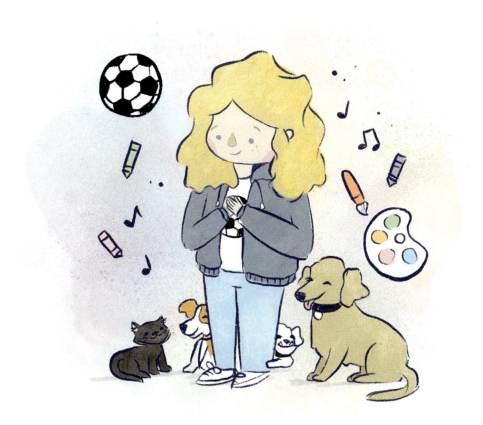

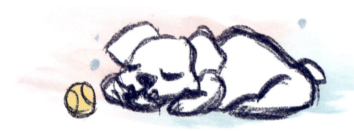

From the Author

Long before I was formally diagnosed with Generalized Anxiety Disorder, I was often seen as the overly sensitive child, teased for taking after my paternal grandmother who "worried enough for everyone she knew." I was riddled with fear, primarily the phobia of dying, and coped with my angst through physically punishing myself by biting my hands until I left marks on them.

As I grew older, I learned how to suppress my "worries" so that others wouldn't find me to be too different, or too needy. I became super compliant by following all the rules and using all my manners. I was seen as a helper in the classroom, and a sweet and mild tempered child at home. All the while, I was fighting a silent battle within.

When I had my first panic attack at age 20, I could no longer move through life in denial that something was making my brain operate differently than others'. I was finally connected to professionals who were able to identify my disorder, and assure me that I wasn't broken. My brain chemistry was simply unique. I began to learn the skills necessary to function in partnership with my anxiety.

After our first daughter, Delilah (DJ for short), was born in 2009, within only a few years of her life, we were able to identify her own anxious tendencies. She was easily startled, had massive separation anxiety (that never decreased), and refused to sleep alone. As DJ grew older, she developed her own phobias, grew very selective about her friendships, preferred to stay at home, and often refused to engage in new experiences. By 5 years old, DJ started to protest preschool, and began exhibiting signs of panic.

It has been through DJ's own work in therapy, home resources, relationships with her school counselors and trusted teachers, that she has found confidence and empowerment in knowing she can affectively navigate life despite having anxiety. She knows how to call upon her Truth Queen in the most vulnerable of times.

Through my transition from the corporate world, to stay-at-home parenting, and into teaching, I have encountered countless children with anxiety. Sometimes it displays in ways similar to mine and DJ's, and other times it shows up as classroom disruption. Maybe it looks like non-compliance in group settings, or tantrums when things get too loud. Maybe it looks like frequent trips to the bathroom, or even frequent absences. Anxious children are brilliant in their ability to channel their nervous energy into action. As an educator, I know it's not always easy for you, but I promise you that if you look a little deeper, you might just see your student's difficult behavior as a cry to feel safe.

This book is for you. Together, DJ and I wrote this book from personal experience, and with the hope that it would be a conversation starter. Whether you're the parent of an anxious child who is just starting to figure this whole thing out, or you're a teacher who is entrusted with the lives of countless children, we want this book and the following worksheets to be a resource for you. Finally, if you're a child with anxiety, we desperately want you to know that you are not alone. You have a Truth Queen/King within you, and you will learn how to call upon their voice when you need it most. You got this.

- Gina Perkins, Co-Author

What are some of the things that make you most proud of you?
Revisit this list whenever you're feeling blue.

1.
2.
3.
4.
5.
6.
7.
8.
9.
10.

Remember, you are perfect just the way you are.
YOU were born to be a star!

Use each box below to write down any Story Bugs living inside your brain.

Once you're done, cut them out and place the Story Bugs inside your Worry Box.

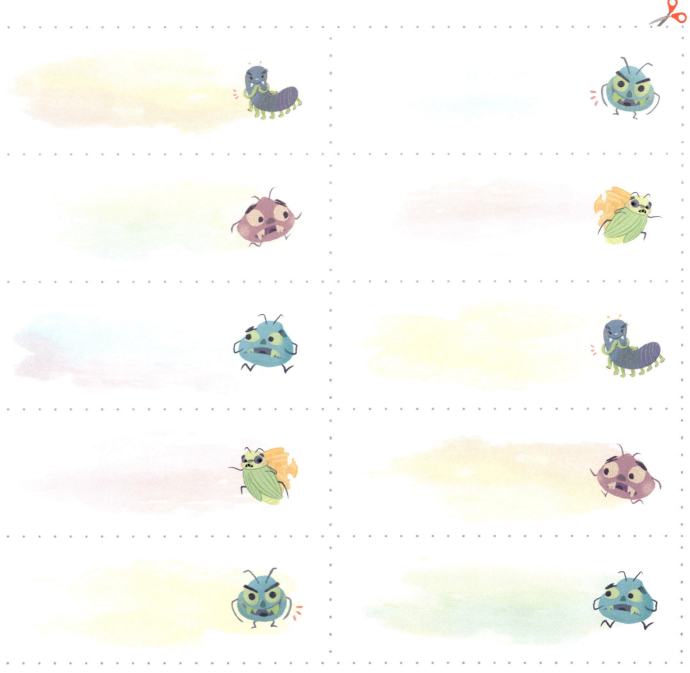

Make Your Own Mini Worry Box!

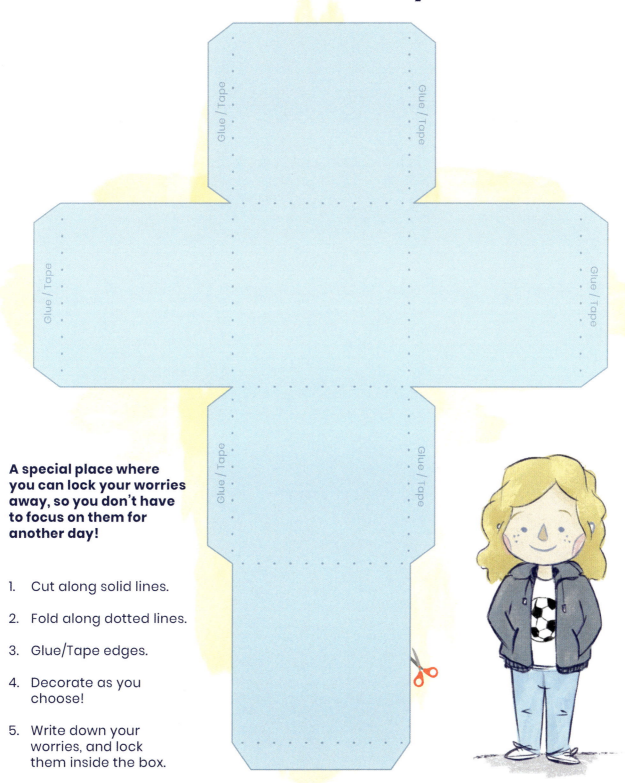

A special place where you can lock your worries away, so you don't have to focus on them for another day!

1. Cut along solid lines.
2. Fold along dotted lines.
3. Glue/Tape edges.
4. Decorate as you choose!
5. Write down your worries, and lock them inside the box.

Made in the USA
San Bernardino, CA
21 November 2019

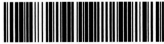